THE ESSENTIAL RENAL DIET COOKBOOK FOR BEGINNERS

20 Delicious & Easy-to-Make Low Sodium, Low Potassium and Low Phosphorus Recipes for a Healthy Kidney and Avoid Dialysis with a 30-Days Meal Plan.

Wellness Words

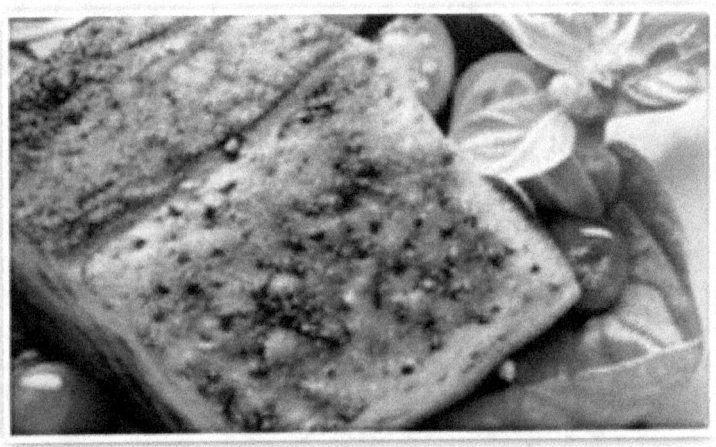

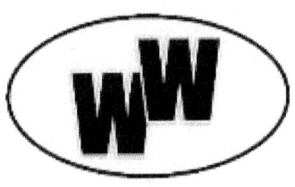

TABLE OF CONTENTS

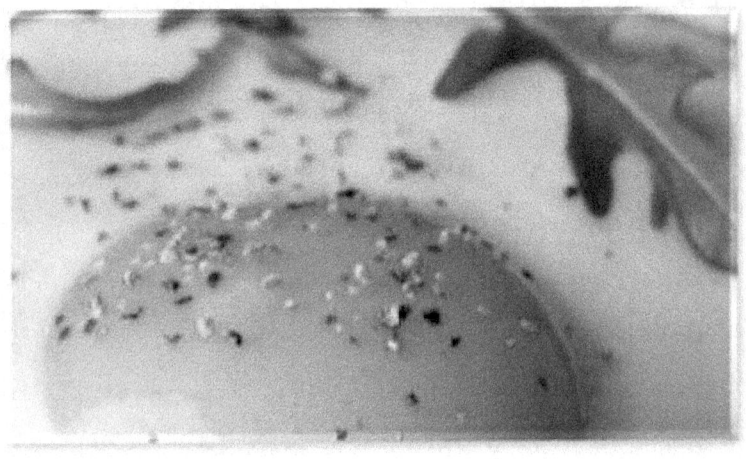

INTRODUCTION

Williams, a middle-aged guy, has been dealing with serious renal difficulties for some years. Despite several tries at various therapies and diets, his health remained dire, and hope was fading. In his frantic hunt for a solution, he came upon a glimmer of light - **THE ESSENTIAL RENAL DIET COOKBOOK FOR BEGINNERS.**

Williams was intrigued by the idea of a diet designed exclusively for people with renal illness and decided to give it a try. Following the recipes and directions in the cookbook, he set off on a voyage. To his delight, the dishes were not only simple to create but also contained easily available components. His renal function improved so quickly that he was shocked and relieved.

Williams was obliged to share the revolutionary secret of The Essential Renal Diet Cookbook for Beginners with his circle of friends and family after being overjoyed by the favorable outcomes. He enthusiastically related his encounter with the book, encouraged others to investigate its potential advantages.

Williams held The Essential Renal Diet Cookbook for Beginners close to him, utilizing it as a loyal friend in sustaining his newfound health. Recognizing the blessing of this seemingly miraculous cure, he was moved by a desire to extend its advantages to as many people as possible.

The Essential Renal Diet Cookbook for Beginners is a thorough handbook that provides helpful insights into creating meals designed to fulfill the nutritional needs of persons suffering from renal disease.

This cookbook not only gives advice on cooking healthy and nutritious meals, but it also aids individuals in developing a well-balanced diet according to their own needs. It has a selection of delectable recipes that allow users to easily create healthful meals in the comfort of their own homes.

The recipes, which emphasize low-sodium and low-protein alternatives, are meticulously created to encourage improved kidney function. Furthermore, the cookbook contains instructions for producing easy yet delectable foods that contribute to heart-healthy eating. Individuals may use this cookbook to properly control their kidney health via the transformational power of eating.

What Exactly Is The Renal Diet?

A Renal Diet is a tailored dietary regimen targeted at protecting kidney health. This diet is tailored to each individual's medical history, taking into account the kind and amount of renal illness they may have. It is characterized by low levels of sodium, potassium, phosphorus, and protein. It may also need extra changes, such as limiting fluid consumption.

The major goal of a renal diet is to reduce the stress on the kidneys by minimizing the presence of waste and toxins in the body. This is accomplished by reducing protein consumption while preserving electrolyte balances such as sodium, potassium, and phosphorus.

When starting a renal diet, it is critical to speak with a nutritionist or doctor to verify that the diet meets the individual's unique needs. It should include a wide variety of meals, including fruits and vegetables, to ensure enough nutrition and avoid any deficiencies.

Food limits in a renal diet usually target red meat, dairy products, processed meals, and salt and potassium-rich foods. Protein consumption is likewise restricted, since an excess might strain the kidneys.

A healthy lifestyle, in addition to food changes, is essential. Regular exercise, quitting smoking, and limiting alcohol use all help to overall kidney health.

Individuals may actively protect their kidneys by following a renal diet and integrating positive lifestyle modifications, lowering the probability of kidney disease consequences.

GUIDELINES ON FOOD CHOICES FOR KIDNEY HEALTH

Living with chronic renal disease does not have to limit your capacity to live a normal life. Adopting a healthy and well-balanced diet can help to manage the illness and avoid its development. Dietary choices might differ depending on whether a person is on dialysis or has chronic renal disease.

Based on your unique needs, your doctor may propose changes to your protein intake, hydration consumption, and mineral or electrolyte limits. Here are some critical guidelines for those with kidney problems:

Foods to Eat

Low-Sodium Foods: Choose fresh fruits and vegetables as well as low-sodium lean meats. This option reduces the risk of high blood pressure and water retention.

High-Fiber Foods: Include foods high in fiber, such as whole grains, legumes, and vegetables, to support good digestion and nutrient absorption. This can assist relieve renal tension.

Low-Potassium Foods: Limit your potassium consumption by eliminating high-potassium foods such as bananas, potatoes, and tomatoes. This is especially important for people who have renal difficulties since potassium clearance may be impaired.

Low-Phosphorus Alternatives: Limit consumption of high-phosphorus foods such as dairy products and red meat, as poor kidney function may hinder phosphorus removal.

Protein-Rich Foods: Maintain muscular health and strength by eating protein-rich, low-phosphorus foods like fish, eggs, and lean meats.

Calcium-Rich Foods: Promote bone health by consuming calcium-rich foods such as dairy products, tofu, and leafy greens in your diet.

Foods to Avoid

Processed Foods: Avoid processed foods, which frequently include high levels of salt, potassium, and phosphorus, which can be harmful to those who have renal issues.

Canned Foods: Because of their high salt and phosphorus levels, canned foods should be avoided by people with renal problems.

High-Sodium Foods: Limit your consumption of high-sodium foods such as processed meats, canned soups, and pickled foods to reduce your risk of high blood pressure and water retention.

High-Potassium Foods: Limit your intake of high-potassium foods such as bananas, potatoes, and tomatoes, as high potassium levels can be harmful.

High-Phosphorus Foods: Limit your diet of high-phosphorus foods such dairy products, red meat, and processed meals to reduce your risk of higher phosphorus levels.

Alcohol: Alcohol should be used with caution since it can cause dehydration and may be dangerous to people who have renal issues.

These dietary advice, when tailored with the assistance of a healthcare practitioner, help greatly to preserving kidney health and decreasing difficulties associated with renal disease.

20 DELECTABLE RENAL DIET DISHES

Slow Cooker Lentil Soup

- **Prep Time:** 15 minutes
- **Cook Time:** 4 hours
- **Ingredients:**
  - 2 tablespoons olive oil
  - 1 onion, diced
  - 2 cloves garlic, minced
  - 1 teaspoon dried oregano
  - 1 teaspoon ground cumin
  - 6 cups vegetable broth
  - 1 (14-oz) can diced tomatoes
  - 1 cup dried lentils, rinsed
  - 2 tablespoons fresh parsley, finely minced
  - Salt and pepper, to taste

Method:

1. Warm olive oil in a pan over medium heat.
2. Sauté onion until softened (about 5 minutes).

3. Add cumin, oregano, and garlic; cook for 1 minute.

4. Transfer the mixture to a slow cooker.

5. Add vegetable broth, tomatoes, lentils, and parsley; stir to combine.

6. Cook on low for 4 hours until lentils are tender.

7. Season with salt and pepper.

Baked Salmon with Avocado Salsa

- **Prep Time:** 10 minutes

- **Cook Time:** 10 minutes

- **Ingredients:**

    - 4 (5-oz) salmon fillets

    - 2 tablespoons olive oil

    - 1 ripe avocado, diced

    - 1/4 cup fresh cilantro, finely minced

    - 2 tablespoons fresh lime juice

    - Salt and pepper, to taste

Method:

1. Preheat oven to 425°F.

2. Grease and line a baking sheet with foil.

3. Place salmon fillets on the baking sheet.

4. Drizzle with olive oil, season with salt and pepper.

5. Bake for 10 minutes until salmon is cooked.

6. In a bowl, combine diced avocado, cilantro, and lime juice.

7. Serve salmon topped with avocado salsa.

Grilled Tuna with Avocado Salad

- **Prep Time:** 10 minutes
- **Cook Time:** 8-10 minutes
- **Ingredients:**
    - 2 (4-oz) tuna steaks
    - 2 tablespoons olive oil
    - 1 ripe avocado, diced
    - 1/4 cup fresh parsley, finely minced
    - 2 tablespoons fresh lemon juice
    - Salt and pepper, to taste

Method:

1. Preheat grill or grill pan to medium-high heat.

2. Brush tuna steaks with olive oil, season with salt and pepper.

3. Grill for 4-5 minutes per side until tuna is cooked.

4. In a bowl, combine diced avocado, parsley, and lemon juice.

5. Serve tuna topped with avocado salad.

Baked Cod with Herbs

- **Prep Time:** 10 minutes

- **Cook Time:** 10 minutes

- **Ingredients:**

  - 4 (4-oz) cod fillets

  - 2 tablespoons olive oil

  - 2 tablespoons fresh parsley, finely minced

  - 2 tablespoons fresh thyme, finely minced

  - Salt and pepper, to taste

Method:

1. Preheat oven to 425°F.

2. Grease and line a baking sheet with foil.

3. Place cod fillets on the baking sheet.

4. Drizzle with olive oil, sprinkle with parsley, thyme, salt, and pepper.

5. Bake for 10 minutes until cod is cooked through.

Grilled Eggplant with Balsamic Glaze

- **Prep Time:** 10 minutes
- **Cook Time:** 8-10 minutes
- **Ingredients:**
    - 2 large eggplants, cut into 1/2-inch slices
    - 2 tablespoons olive oil
    - 2 tablespoons balsamic vinegar
    - 2 tablespoons honey
    - Salt and pepper, to taste

Method:

1. Preheat grill or grill pan to medium-high heat.

2. Brush eggplant slices with olive oil, season with salt and pepper.

3. Grill for 3-4 minutes per side until eggplant is tender.

4. In a saucepan, bring balsamic vinegar and honey to a boil, then simmer until thickened.

5. Serve grilled eggplant topped with balsamic glaze.

Baked Sliced Apples

- **Prep Time:** 10 minutes
- **Cook Time:** 25-30 minutes
- **Ingredients:**
    - 4 large apples, cored and sliced
    - 2 tablespoons olive oil
    - 2 tablespoons brown sugar
    - 2 teaspoons ground cinnamon
    - 2 tablespoons chopped walnuts
    - 2 tablespoons raisins

Method:

1. Preheat oven to 375°F.
2. Grease and line a baking sheet with foil.
3. Arrange apple slices in a single layer on the baking sheet.
4. Drizzle with olive oil, sprinkle with brown sugar, cinnamon, walnuts, and raisins.
5. Bake for 25-30 minutes until apples are soft.

Roasted Brussels Sprouts

- **Prep Time:** 10 minutes
- **Cook Time:** 25-30 minutes
- **Ingredients:**
  - 2 lb. Brussels sprouts, trimmed and halved
  - 2 tablespoons olive oil
  - 2 cloves garlic, minced
  - Salt and pepper, to taste

Method:

1. Preheat oven to 425°F.
2. Grease and line a baking sheet with foil.
3. Arrange Brussels sprouts in a single layer on the baking sheet.
4. Drizzle with olive oil, sprinkle with garlic, salt, and pepper.
5. Bake for 25-30 minutes until Brussels sprouts are tender.

Baked Eggplant with Tomatoes

- **Prep Time:** 10 minutes
- **Cook Time:** 25-30 minutes
- **Ingredients:**
    - 1 large eggplant, cut into 1-inch cubes
    - 2 tablespoons olive oil
    - 2 cups cherry tomatoes
    - 2 tablespoons fresh basil, finely minced
    - Salt and pepper, to taste

Method:

1. Preheat oven to 425°F.
2. Grease and line a baking sheet with foil.
3. Arrange eggplant cubes and cherry tomatoes in a single layer on the baking sheet.
4. Drizzle with olive oil, sprinkle with basil, salt, and pepper.
5. Bake for 25-30 minutes until eggplant is tender.

Roasted Cauliflower with Parmesan

- **Prep Time:** 10 minutes
- **Cook Time:** 25-30 minutes
- **Ingredients:**
  - 1 head cauliflower, cut into florets
  - 2 tablespoons olive oil
  - 1/2 cup grated Parmesan cheese
  - Salt and pepper, to taste

Method:

1. Preheat oven to 425°F.
2. Grease and line a baking sheet with foil.
3. Arrange cauliflower florets in a single layer on the baking sheet.
4. Drizzle with olive oil, sprinkle with Parmesan cheese, salt, and pepper.
5. Bake for 25-30 minutes until cauliflower is tender.

Baked Tofu with Soy Sauce

- **Prep Time:** 10 minutes
- **Cook Time:** 25-30 minutes
- **Ingredients:**
    - 1 lb. extra-firm tofu, cut into cubes
    - 2 tablespoons olive oil
    - 1/4 cup low-sodium soy sauce
    - 1 teaspoon sesame oil
    - 2 cloves garlic, minced
    - 2 tablespoons fresh ginger, grated
    - Salt and pepper, to taste

Method:

1. Preheat oven to 425°F.
2. Grease and line a baking sheet with foil.
3. Place tofu cubes on the baking sheet.
4. In a small bowl, whisk together soy sauce, sesame oil, garlic, and ginger.
5. Drizzle the marinade over the tofu cubes and toss to coat.
6. Bake for 25-30 minutes until tofu is golden brown.

Quinoa and Black Bean Salad

- **Prep Time:** 15 minutes
- **Cook Time:** 15 minutes
- **Ingredients:**
    - 1 cup uncooked quinoa
    - 2 cups vegetable broth
    - 2 tablespoons olive oil
    - 1 (14-oz) can black beans, drained and rinsed
    - 1 red bell pepper, diced
    - 1/4 cup fresh cilantro, finely minced
    - 2 tablespoons fresh lime juice
    - Salt and pepper, to taste

Method:

1. In a medium saucepan, bring quinoa and vegetable broth to a boil.

2. Reduce heat to low, cover, and simmer until all the liquid has been absorbed (about 15 minutes).

3. Remove from heat and fluff with a fork.

4. In a large bowl, combine quinoa, black beans, bell pepper, cilantro, and lime juice.

5. Drizzle with olive oil and season with salt and pepper.

Lentil and Spinach Curry

- **Prep Time:** 10 minutes
- **Cook Time:** 25-30 minutes
- **Ingredients:**
    - 2 tablespoons olive oil
    - 1 onion, diced
    - 2 cloves garlic, minced
    - 2 teaspoons curry powder
    - 2 cups vegetable broth
    - 1 (14-oz) can diced tomatoes
    - 1 cup dried lentils, rinsed
    - 2 cups baby spinach
    - Salt and pepper, to taste

Method:

1. Heat olive oil in a large saucepan over medium heat.

2. Add diced onion and sauté for 5 minutes until tender.

3. Stir in garlic and curry powder; cook for an additional 1 minute.

4. Add vegetable broth, diced tomatoes, and lentils; bring to a boil.

5. Reduce heat to low, cover, and simmer for about 20 minutes or until lentils are tender.

6. Stir in baby spinach and cook until wilted (about 2 minutes).

7. Season with salt and pepper to taste.

Grilled Halibut with Lemon and Parsley

- **Prep Time:** 10 minutes

- **Cook Time:** 10 minutes

- **Ingredients:**

    - 4 (4-oz) halibut fillets

    - 2 tablespoons olive oil

    - 2 tablespoons fresh parsley, finely minced

    - 2 tablespoons fresh lemon juice

    - Salt and pepper, to taste

Method:

1. Preheat grill or grill pan to medium-high heat.

2. Brush halibut fillets with olive oil and season with salt and pepper.

3. Grill for 5 minutes per side or until halibut is cooked through.

4. Remove from heat and top with minced parsley and lemon juice.

Grilled Shrimp Skewers

- **Prep Time:** 15 minutes

- **Cook Time:** 6 minutes

- **Ingredients:**

    - 1 lb. large shrimp, peeled and deveined

    - 2 tablespoons olive oil

    - 1 teaspoon smoked paprika

    - 1/2 teaspoon garlic powder

    - Salt and pepper, to taste

    - 8 (8-inch) bamboo skewers, soaked in water

Method:

1. Preheat grill or grill pan to medium-high heat.

2. Thread 4 shrimp onto each soaked skewer.

3. Brush skewers with olive oil and season with smoked paprika, garlic powder, salt, and pepper.

4. Grill for 2-3 minutes per side or until shrimp are cooked through.

Broiled Tilapia with Garlic and Parsley

- **Prep Time:** 7 minutes
- **Cook Time:** 7-8 minutes
- **Ingredients:**
    - 4 (4-oz) tilapia fillets
    - 2 tablespoons olive oil
    - 2 tablespoons fresh parsley, finely minced
    - 2 cloves garlic, minced
    - Salt and pepper, to taste

Method:

1. Preheat broiler to high heat.
2. Grease and line a baking sheet with foil.
3. Place tilapia fillets on the baking sheet.
4. Drizzle with olive oil and sprinkle with parsley, minced garlic, salt, and pepper.
5. Broil for 7-8 minutes or until tilapia is cooked through.

Poached Eggs with Spinach

- **Prep Time:** 5 minutes
- **Cook Time:** 7-8 minutes
- **Ingredients:**
    - 2 tablespoons olive oil
    - 2 cloves garlic, minced
    - 2 cups baby spinach
    - 4 large eggs
    - Salt and pepper, to taste

Method:

1. Heat olive oil in a large pan over medium heat.
2. Add minced garlic and cook for 1 minute.
3. Add spinach and cook until wilted.
4. Reduce heat to low and crack eggs into the pan.
5. Cover the pan and cook until eggs are set (about 4-5 minutes).
6. Season with salt and pepper.

Baked Zucchini with Parmesan

- **Prep Time:** 10 minutes
- **Cook Time:** 15-20 minutes
- **Ingredients:**
  - 4 small zucchinis, sliced into 1/4-inch rounds
  - 2 tablespoons olive oil
  - 1/2 cup grated Parmesan cheese
  - 2 tablespoons fresh parsley, finely minced
  - Salt and pepper, to taste

Method:

1. Preheat oven to 425°F.
2. Grease and line a baking sheet with foil.
3. Arrange zucchini rounds in a single layer on the baking sheet.
4. Drizzle with olive oil and sprinkle with Parmesan cheese, parsley, salt, and pepper.
5. Bake for 15-20 minutes or until zucchini is tender.

Steamed Broccoli with Lemon and Garlic

- **Prep Time:** 5 minutes

- **Cook Time:** 5-7 minutes

- **Ingredients:**

    - 2 heads broccoli, cut into florets

    - 2 tablespoons olive oil

    - 2 cloves garlic, minced

    - 2 tablespoons fresh lemon juice

    - Salt and pepper, to taste

Method:

1. Bring 1 inch of water to a boil in a large pot.

2. Place broccoli in a steamer basket and put it in the pot.

3. Cover and steam for 5-7 minutes until broccoli is tender.

4. Remove from heat and toss with olive oil, minced garlic, lemon juice, salt, and pepper.

Roasted Asparagus with Parmesan

- **Prep Time:** 5 minutes
- **Cook Time:** 10-15 minutes
- **Ingredients:**
  - 2 bunches asparagus, trimmed
  - 2 tablespoons olive oil
  - 1/2 cup grated Parmesan cheese
  - Salt and pepper, to taste

Method:

1. Preheat oven to 425°F.

2. Grease and line a baking sheet with foil.

3. Arrange asparagus in a single layer on the baking sheet.

4. Drizzle with olive oil and sprinkle with Parmesan cheese, salt, and pepper.

5. Bake for 10-15 minutes or until asparagus is tender.

Baked Sweet Potato Fries

- **Prep Time:** 5 minutes

- **Cook Time:** 20-25 minutes

- **Ingredients:**

    - 2 large sweet potatoes, sliced into matchsticks

    - 2 tablespoons olive oil

    - Salt and pepper, to taste

Method:

1. Preheat oven to 425°F.

2. Grease and line a baking sheet with foil.

3. Arrange sweet potato matchsticks in a single layer on the baking sheet.

4. Drizzle with olive oil and sprinkle with salt and pepper.

5. Bake for 20-25 minutes or until sweet potatoes are tender.

30 DAYS MEAL PLAN

A complete 30-day meal plan that promotes kidney health while providing a delectable culinary experience. Each day is carefully chosen to include a different combination of breakfast, lunch, and supper meals, offering a varied and delectable trip through renal-friendly food.

This cookbook offers a balanced and tasty approach to keeping a healthy renal diet, with recipes ranging from the flavorful Baked Salmon with Avocado Salsa to the nutritious Slow Cooker Lentil Soup. Enjoy the diversity, taste the flavors, and embark on a nutritious gastronomic journey for optimal kidney health.

Day 1:
- **Breakfast:** Poached Eggs with Spinach
- **Lunch:** Quinoa and Black Bean Salad
- **Dinner:** Grilled Halibut with Lemon and Parsley

Day 2:
- **Breakfast:** Baked Sliced Apples
- **Lunch:** Roasted Brussels Sprouts
- **Dinner:** Baked Tofu with Soy Sauce

Day 3:
- **Breakfast:** Lentil and Spinach Curry
- **Lunch:** Steamed Broccoli with Lemon and Garlic
- **Dinner:** Baked Cod with Herbs

Day 4:
- **Breakfast:** Baked Zucchini with Parmesan
- **Lunch:** Roasted Asparagus with Parmesan
- **Dinner:** Grilled Shrimp Skewers

Day 5:
- **Breakfast:** Baked Sweet Potato Fries
- **Lunch:** Slow Cooker Lentil Soup
- **Dinner:** Baked Eggplant with Tomatoes

Day 6:
- **Breakfast:** Roasted Chickpeas with Garlic and Rosemary
- **Lunch:** Grilled Tuna with Avocado Salad
- **Dinner:** Broiled Tilapia with Garlic and Parsley

Day 7:
- **Breakfast:** Baked Salmon with Avocado Salsa
- **Lunch:** Roasted Cauliflower with Parmesan
- **Dinner:** Grilled Eggplant with Balsamic Glaze

Day 8:
- **Breakfast:** Baked Salmon with Rosemary and Thyme
- **Lunch:** Quinoa and Black Bean Salad
- **Dinner:** Lentil and Spinach Curry

Day 9:

- **Breakfast:** Grilled Halibut with Lemon and Parsley
- **Lunch:** Baked Cod with Herbs
- **Dinner:** Baked Sweet Potato Fries

Day 10:

- **Breakfast:** Roasted Asparagus with Parmesan
- **Lunch:** Baked Tofu with Soy Sauce
- **Dinner:** Grilled Shrimp Skewers

Day 11:

- **Breakfast:** Lentil and Spinach Curry
- **Lunch:** Baked Eggplant with Tomatoes
- **Dinner:** Roasted Chickpeas with Garlic and Rosemary

Day 12:

- **Breakfast:** Baked Zucchini with Parmesan
- **Lunch:** Grilled Tuna with Avocado Salad
- **Dinner:** Steamed Broccoli with Lemon and Garlic

Day 13:

- **Breakfast:** Baked Sliced Apples
- **Lunch:** Slow Cooker Lentil Soup
- **Dinner:** Broiled Tilapia with Garlic and Parsley

Day 14:
- **Breakfast:** Grilled Eggplant with Balsamic Glaze
- **Lunch:** Baked Salmon with Avocado Salsa
- **Dinner:** Roasted Cauliflower with Parmesan

Day 15:
- **Breakfast:** Poached Eggs with Spinach
- **Lunch:** Quinoa and Black Bean Salad
- **Dinner:** Roasted Brussels Sprouts

Day 16:
- **Breakfast:** Baked Tofu with Soy Sauce
- **Lunch:** Grilled Shrimp Skewers
- **Dinner:** Lentil and Spinach Curry

Day 17:
- **Breakfast:** Broiled Tilapia with Garlic and Parsley
- **Lunch:** Baked Eggplant with Tomatoes
- **Dinner:** Grilled Tuna with Avocado Salad

Day 18:
- **Breakfast:** Roasted Cauliflower with Parmesan
- **Lunch:** Baked Sweet Potato Fries
- **Dinner:** Grilled Halibut with Lemon and Parsley

Day 19:
- **Breakfast:** Roasted Chickpeas with Garlic and Rosemary
- **Lunch:** Steamed Broccoli with Lemon and Garlic
- **Dinner:** Quinoa and Black Bean Salad

Day 20:
- **Breakfast:** Baked Salmon with Avocado Salsa
- **Lunch:** Roasted Brussels Sprouts
- **Dinner:** Baked Zucchini with Parmesan

Day 21:
- **Breakfast:** Baked Cod with Herbs
- **Lunch:** Slow Cooker Lentil Soup
- **Dinner:** Baked Sliced Apples

Day 22:
- **Breakfast:** Roasted Asparagus with Parmesan
- **Lunch:** Grilled Eggplant with Balsamic Glaze
- **Dinner:** Baked Salmon with Rosemary and Thyme

Day 23:
- **Breakfast:** Grilled Shrimp Skewers
- **Lunch:** Lentil and Spinach Curry
- **Dinner:** Baked Sweet Potato Fries

Day 24:
- **Breakfast:** Grilled Tuna with Avocado Salad
- **Lunch:** Roasted Chickpeas with Garlic and Rosemary
- **Dinner:** Broiled Tilapia with Garlic and Parsley

Day 25:
- **Breakfast:** Quinoa and Black Bean Salad
- **Lunch:** Grilled Halibut with Lemon and Parsley
- **Dinner:** Baked Zucchini with Parmesan

Day 26:
- **Breakfast:** Baked Eggplant with Tomatoes
- **Lunch:** Baked Sliced Apples
- **Dinner:** Steamed Broccoli with Lemon and Garlic

Day 27:
- **Breakfast:** Slow Cooker Lentil Soup
- **Lunch:** Roasted Brussels Sprouts
- **Dinner:** Baked Cod with Herbs

Day 28:
- **Breakfast:** Roasted Cauliflower with Parmesan
- **Lunch:** Baked Tofu with Soy Sauce
- **Dinner:** Grilled Shrimp Skewers

Day 29:
- **Breakfast:** Baked Sweet Potato Fries
- **Lunch:** Baked Salmon with Rosemary and Thyme
- **Dinner:** Grilled Eggplant with Balsamic Glaze

Day 30:
- **Breakfast:** Roasted Asparagus with Parmesan
- **Lunch:** Grilled Halibut with Lemon and Parsley
- **Dinner:** Poached Eggs with Spinach

CONCLUSION

The route to renal fitness has never been more delectable and accessible, due to "The Essential Renal Diet Cookbook for Beginners." This culinary masterwork surpasses the boundaries of typical cookbooks, providing a lifeline to people seeking not only food but a wonderful marriage of health and taste.

This indispensable handbook emerges as a trusted friend, deftly revealing the subtleties of the renal diet. Its beauty resides not just in the delectable meals, but also in the profound insight it conveys about supporting kidneys via culinary artistry.

The cookbook is more than just a compilation of recipes; it's a symphony of tastes geared to renal wellness. This cookbook transcends its label, becoming a culinary compass for various palates, whether you're a newbie ready to adopt a kidney-friendly lifestyle or a seasoned practitioner looking for culinary inspiration.

What distinguishes this cookbook is its natural capacity to empower. It converts the seemingly difficult renal diet into a delectable gastronomic adventure. Every page exudes the enthusiasm of someone truly involved in your health journey, from clear directions to morsels of nutritional advice.

"The Essential Renal Diet Cookbook for Beginners" is more than simply a recipe book; it's a manifesto of tasty options that improve health. It's a testimony to perseverance and a reminder that taking responsibility of your health can be a delectable adventure.

With its pages transformed into culinary paintings, this cookbook is an homage to the delight of eating well, a must-have for everyone who appreciates the creativity of a health-conscious kitchen.

REDUCE THE STRESS ON THE KIDNEY AND MINIMIZE THE PRESENCE OF WASTE AND TOXINS IN THE BODY!!!